Quick Fix Your Sex Life

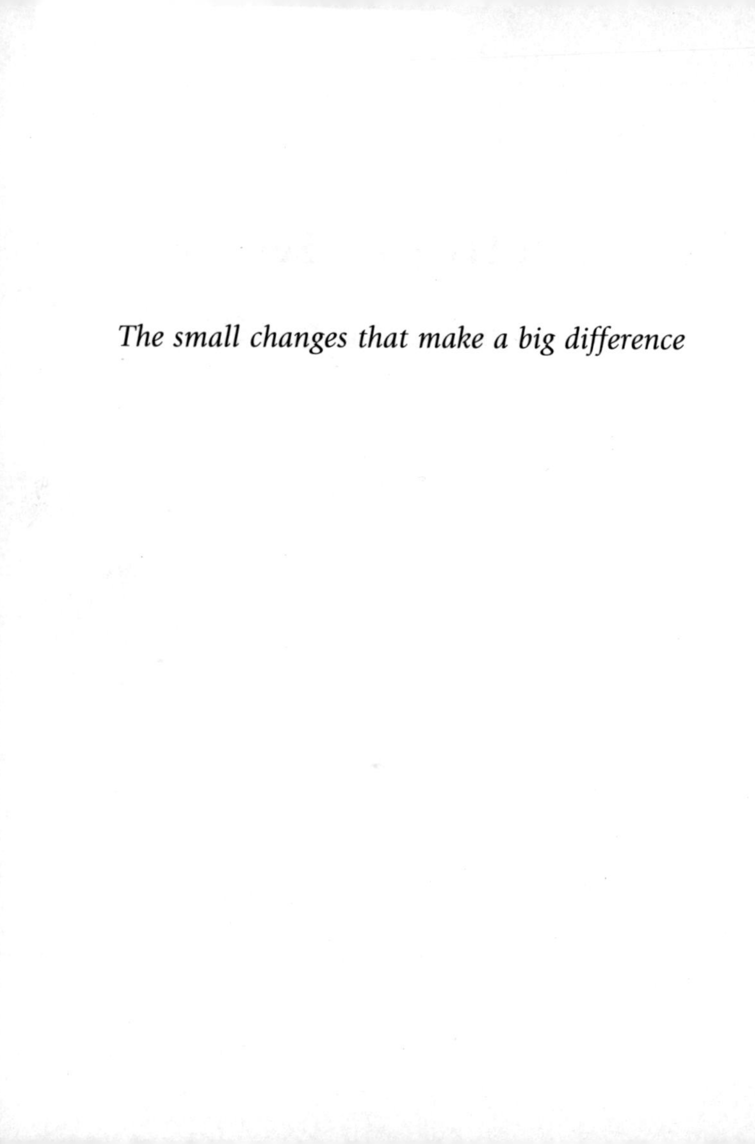

The small changes that make a big difference

Quick Fix Your Sex Life

Judith Verity

How To Books

Published by How To Books Ltd,
3 Newtec Place, Magdalen Road,
Oxford OX4 1RE. United Kingdom.
Tel: (01865) 793806. Fax: (01865) 248780.
email: info@howtobooks.co.uk
http://www.howtobooks.co.uk

British Library Cataloguing in Publication Data.

A catalogue record for this book is available from the British Library.

Cover design by Shireen Nathoo Design, London
Cover illustration by Roger Langridge
Cartoons by Grizelda Grizlingham

Produced for How To Books by Deer Park Productions
Design and Typeset by Shireen Nathoo Design, London
Printed and bound in Great Britain

Contents

Introduction

Erotic practices have become diversified. Sex used to be single crop farming, like cotton or wheat; now people raise all kinds of things.

Saul Bellow

There's plenty of information about sex. In fact almost everything seems to have sexual implications. Together with slimming and shopping, it's the most popular subject for articles in women's magazines. It's the main topic in men's magazines too – this time together with sport and shopping.

And that's just the articles. Most of the advertising has a pretty strong sex angle as well. When an ad agency promotes a new product, whether it's a car or a shampoo, the first thing they'll look at is how it might improve your sex life. If it's not sexy it probably won't sell.

And sometimes it's hard to tell the difference between information, advertising and entertainment, because it all looks so sexy. It's safer to assume that most of the in-your-face information about sex that's around at the moment is really a cover for selling you something much more mundane. You may be buying a cleaning product, a movie, a song, or even an image (somebody else's). But you won't be buying a sex life.

The Manuals

So if you can't rely on the glossy magazines for hard advice, what about taking a more academic approach and heading for the library? There are plenty of books with loads of statistics and accurate illustrations, but would you want to be seen reading one on the train? Or keeping one by the side of the bed? When it comes to sex, most people prefer the hands-on approach.

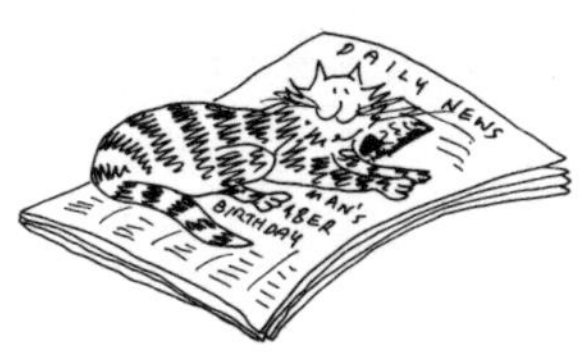

So who do you call to get you up and moving in the right direction? Talking it over seems like the obvious option, but bear in mind that verbal information is usually loaded. Before you take anyone's advice about sex, run a reality check on their hidden agenda.

Ask the Family

Sex is a natural function, a part of family life – so shouldn't you be asking the family if you need advice? You already know it's not that simple.

Assuming your chosen family confidante can cope with the embarrassment of talking about sex in the first place, they'll probably advise you not to do it. After all, if they're older than you they'll be worried about having to pick up the tab if you get AIDS or get pregnant. If they're younger than you they'll be afraid of you having a heart attack or starting another family, and they probably think sex is disgusting at your age anyway.

Friends

Friends of the opposite sex (unless you're gay) are always potential lovers or ex lovers so you can never be sure they don't have a hidden agenda. Friends of the same sex (especially if you're male) will want to make it clear that they have a better sex life than you could ever dream of. And it doesn't matter whether they're telling the truth or not – they certainly aren't going to give you any handy hints about how to do it. Male bonding is great for work and football, but when it comes to sex and cars, biggest is usually best...

Expert Advice

This includes teachers, doctors, social workers, counsellors and everybody else who makes a living out of telling other people how to run their lives. These people are likely to have a political agenda or a product to sell (whether it's a drug or a technique). And they may also have a vested interest in getting you to focus on what's wrong (or what could go wrong) rather than a positive up-and-at-it attitude.

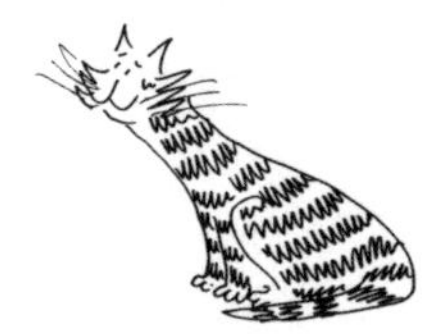

Whatever their angle is, it may not be the best one for you. Remember that sex is a bit like love – little things mean a lot. And this book is about a lot of little things that could make a big difference. All you need is a few minutes to try them out every day and see which ones ring bells for you.

Judith Verity

About the Author

Judith Verity has been in the Life Changing and Personal Development business for thirty years. She now writes for the Human Capital Resources group of trainers, counsellors and musicians.

Judith also works with Pete Cohen on the Lighten Up slimming programme.

To John

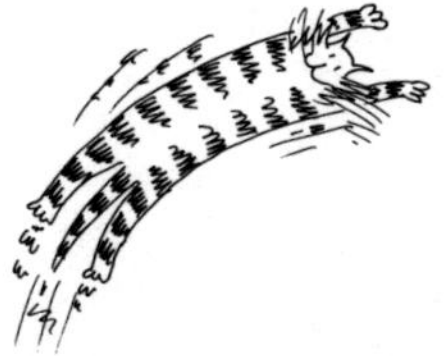

Chapter One

If It Ain't Broke, Don't Fix It

Sex! What is that but Life after all? We're all of us selling sex, because we're all selling life.

ALVIN CHERESKI, SAATCHI & SAATCHI

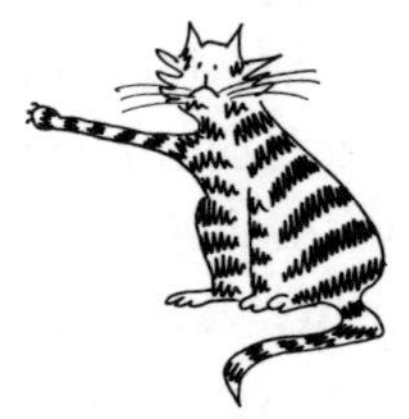

BENEFITS

* Knowing what you want makes it easier to figure out some practical ways of getting it.

BONUS

* Any improvements you make in your sex life, will probably benefit at least one other person – so you aren't being self-indulgent, you're just contributing to the sum of human happiness.

How do you know your sex life needs fixing? And if it does, how do you know what you're looking for? Once a week? Six times a day? Or is it quality rather than quantity you're after?

Choosing a sex life is a pretty recent option. And choice always brings problems with it, as well as pleasures. For the first time in history we can decide what gender we want to be (at a price – hormones and surgery don't come cheap).

And if we can select the body we want to have sex in, surely we ought to have just as much choice about the bodies we have sex *with* as well. And that's just for starters – we also have to figure out when, where and how.

Pete Cohen of Lighten Up told me about a man who turned up to one of his slimming workshops. Apparently this guy didn't look as though he had a weight problem, so Pete was curious and asked him why he was there.

'Slimming groups are cheaper than introduction agencies,' he told Pete, 'and I like big women.'

Now, I'm not saying I approve of that particular strategy. But there's no doubt about it – it's a strategy. That man knew what he wanted and how much he was prepared to pay. If you don't make your own decisions about what you want and how much it's worth, someone else will make those decisions for you. Or nothing will happen at all.

1. Time For a Change?

How do you know your sex life needs fixing?

* Because you can remember when it was better than it is now?
* Because you're getting more complaints than you used to?
* Because it's getting more difficult to find anybody else to do it with?

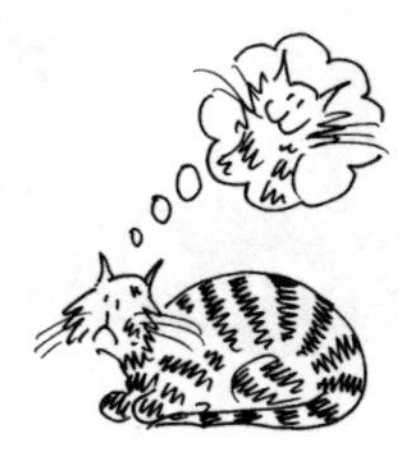

Chapter One

If It Ain't Broke, Don't Fix It

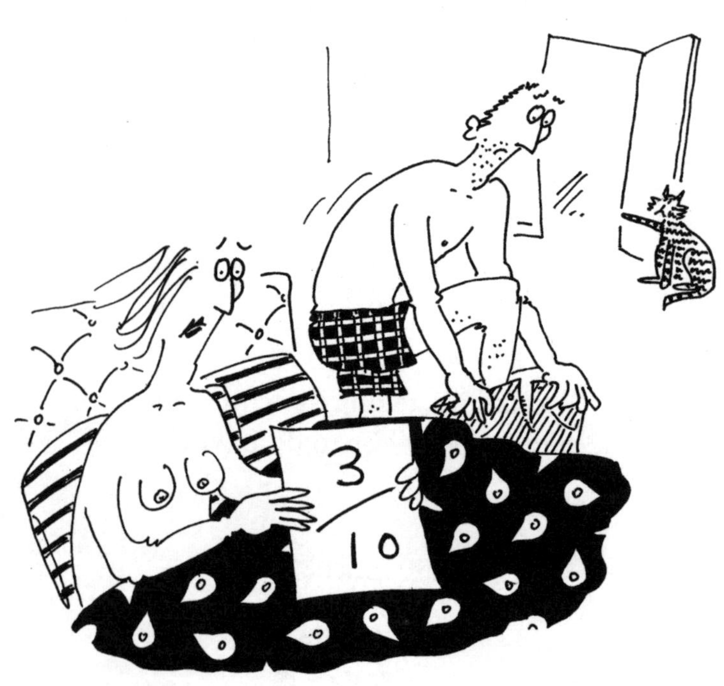

* Because your sex life is unhealthy or illegal?

* Because everybody you know is having more fun than you?

* Because your sex life takes up so much time that you can't get to work in the morning or shop for groceries. (Yes, apparently that *is* a problem for some people!)

Or

* Because your relationship broke up?

* Because you're lonely?

* Because you're bored?

* Because everybody you know *says* they are having more fun than you?

* Because the media and the advertising agencies have sold you the idea that you should be having ecstatically orgasmic sex at least twice a day? And you're not.

What do your answers tell you? Are you sure that you are making your own decision to fix your sex life?

2. What Else is Going On In Your Life?

'What's your name?'
'Ivana Humpalot.'
'Yes, and I want a toilet made out of solid gold but it's just not on the cards now is it?'
AUSTIN POWERS – THE SPY WHO SHAGGED ME

How do you know it's your sex life that needs fixing? However optimistic you are, good quality sex is only going to be one of the hundreds of things you do every day. It's worth taking a look at the broader picture before you jump to conclusions.

Look at the pie chart and mark all the slices which are relevant to you. Anything you do more than once a week will count.

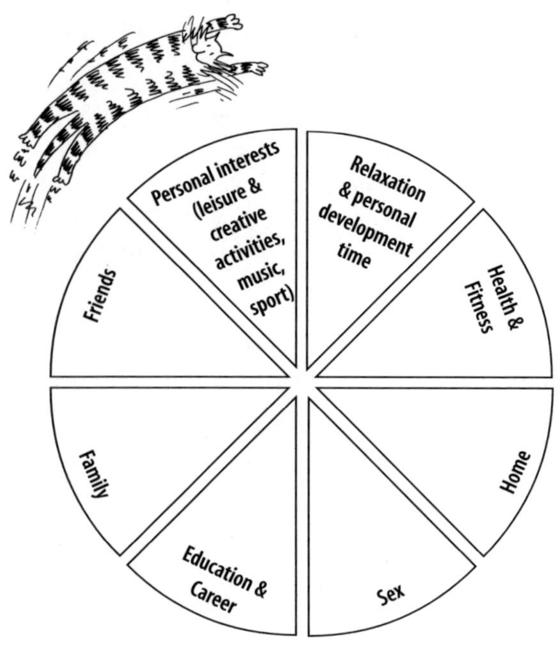
Personal interests (leisure & creative activities, music, sport)
Relaxation & personal development time
Health & Fitness
Home
Sex
Education & Career
Family
Friends

I'm not saying you should have a tick in every slice. If you're young, free and single you might not be visiting your relatives every week or babysitting your nieces and nephews regularly. And if you're a lone parent with not enough hours in the day you might not have much happening in your career or personal interest areas.

The danger signals are when the sex slice is empty or when it's just about the only piece of pie you're getting. In fact, if you fill in half or less of the slices, the chances are you need a bit more balance in your lifestyle. But what's balance got to do with sex? Well, in general sex is better when all the other bits of your life are going well. If sex is all you've got going for you and you lose the urge or your partner leaves, you're going to be bored and depressed (at the very least). But if it's just one of lots of good things you've got in your life, then you can afford some downtime occasionally. Also, the chemicals generated by sex are generated by other sensual activities too (like exercise, eating, and anything that involves smell, taste and touch). So a downturn in the sex department may be regenerated by some of the other things you do.

3. What Do You Want?

If you're still convinced that your sex life really does need fixing, this is the time to be more specific: get into the habit of asking yourself these questions over and over again.

Q What do I want?
A A better sex life.

Q What will that do for me?
A It will take my mind off things / improve my relationships / improve my image or whatever it is for you.

Q So what do I want?
A I want to be happier / get married / have a more exciting social life or whatever it is for you.

Go on looping these questions around until you feel you've got to the bottom of whatever it is. The chances are that your final answer won't be a straight 'I want a better sex life', so you may want to look at some other areas as well.

HOW TO...

* Answer all these questions quickly.
* Make a note of your final answers.

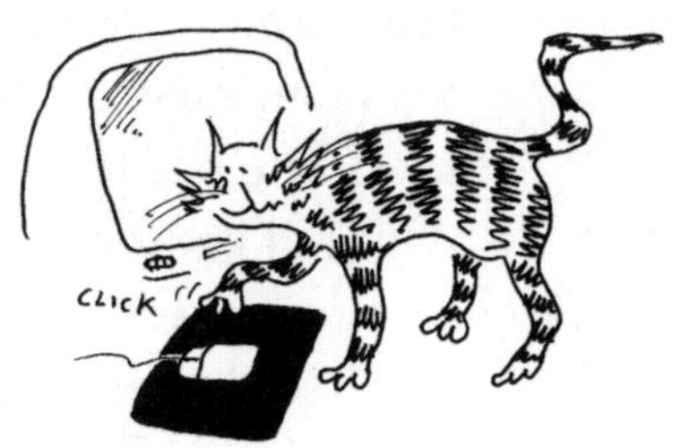

...DO IT

* Go through these questions every day – twice a day if you can manage it – for a week or so.

* At the end of the week, compare your answers. They may be inconsistent – but you'll probably be able to spot a trend.

* Just because your sex life's not so hot at the moment, it doesn't mean your social life has to be on hold as well. Why not get together with another consenting adult and work through this book together? It's more fun when you do it with somebody.

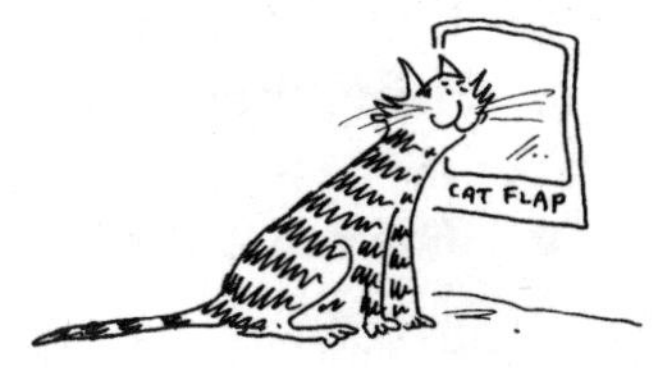
CAT FLAP

Chapter Two

In and Out In the Right Places

I don't know – I'm never there.
DOLLY PARTON

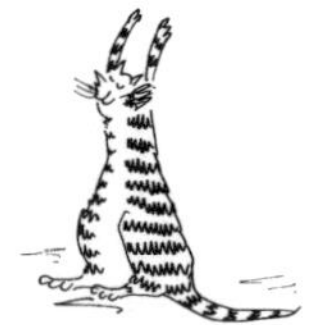

BENEFITS

* If you want to improve your sex life, being there is a good way to start.

* The more you put in, the more you get out.

BONUS

* The sex-life improving ideas in this chapter can be done in the privacy of your own mind while you're commuting or waiting for something to happen. Sure, you could be using the time to fantasise about sex instead, but fantasies are a substitute and this is preparing for the real thing.

If sex is something you do to keep a bargain, earn a living, have a quiet life or solve a problem, then you might well agree with Dolly Parton. She was actually talking about how long it took to do her hair, but if sex is only part of your act rather than who you are, not being there is a perfectly reasonable option.

I called into the local garage last week to collect my car after its MOT. The front desk was empty so I walked through into the workshop where a couple of the mechanics were having tea and reading *The Sun*. The youngest flipped over Page 3 when he saw me and his mate, Kevin, laughed.

The boy blushed and defended himself. 'I bet your girlfriend wouldn't let you stick that picture up over the bed at home.'

Kevin shrugged. 'No way, she couldn't stand the competition.'

'How can a picture of somebody be competition for a real person?'

'They always think you're thinking about somebody else. You just have to pretend you aren't.'

I felt it was time to intervene so I said, 'what do you think women think about when they're having sex.'

'Shopping,' said Kevin. 'At least, Shelley does; after we finished last night she started going on about a new fridge. Mind you, I'd rather have her thinking about kitchen equipment than Brad Pitt's equipment.'

The conversation was getting too depressing so I asked about my car. 'It failed, but then what do you expect, we told you last time, you ought to trade it in.'

1. Testing Neutral

Having a wonderful time; wish I was here.
CALIFORNIAN BUMPER STICKER

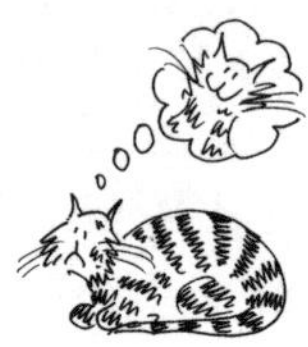

It may not just be a question of sex. Some people hedge their bets when it comes to all of life's most intense experiences – they don't get in too deep because they're afraid they might drown. But if you don't get out of your depth, you'll never learn to swim.

If you don't already know how deep you go, check this.

* Picture yourself coming home. You're walking towards your door, getting out the key, turning it in the lock and stepping inside. Put in as much detail as you can.

* Were you watching from the other side of the street? Or were you actually inside your own body as you walked along?

* Now do this visualisation exercise a couple more times with different ho-hum experiences. Washing up perhaps, or cleaning your teeth. Each time check whether you were in or out of the experience during the replay.

2. Testing Negative

* This time think of something negative – but not a major trauma. Maybe something or somebody who annoyed you; an upsetting incident, a misunderstanding or a situation you couldn't handle.

* Picture yourself going through it all over again, just as it happened.

* When you relive it, what is it like? Are you right in the centre of it, feeling the full effect of the anxiety, anger, frustration or whatever you felt at the time? Or are you standing back watching a movie of the event with yourself as a bit player?

* When you've finished, pick two more of your life's petty irritations and run them through your mind. Check again whether you were in the centre of the storm, or watching from the sidelines.

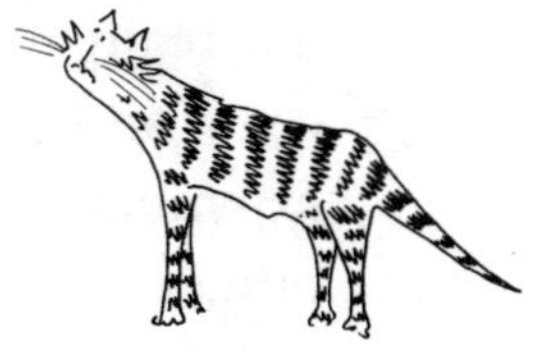

3. Testing Positive

* Now remember the last time you had great sex. Whatever that involved.

* Can you taste it and feel it all over again?

* Were you the star this time? Or in the back row on your own again?

* Find two more times and re-live the moments (or hours). If your sex life has really gone downhill you can cheat and choose another orgasmic experience like a wonderful meal (or a burger if things are really bad). Check, once again, whether you're watching it happen or making it happen.

4. Checking the Results

Bearing in mind that the way you remember events is pretty much the way you experience them, were you

(a) Mostly into it.
(b) Mostly out of it.
(c) Into the good experiences and out of the bad ones.
(d) Into the bad experiences and out of the good ones.
(e) Totally random.

(c) is the ideal way to live your life – distancing yourself from the painful stuff and getting maximum enjoyment out of the good times. But if you already know how to do that, your sex life is probably so wonderful you won't even have time to pick up this book, let alone do the exercises.

The (a)s who pitch right in and experience everything to the full tend to have great sex lives (although they can be dangerous and emotionally harrowing as well). But the (a)s also hit rock bottom when things go wrong – and they go wrong quite often because the (a)s don't usually see problems until it's too late.

The detached (b)s go through life never getting too upset about anything, but never hitting the emotional and physical highs either.

And the (d)s, unfortunately, seem to make up a big proportion of people who have trouble with sex. They just can't get

Chapter Two

In And Out In The Right Places

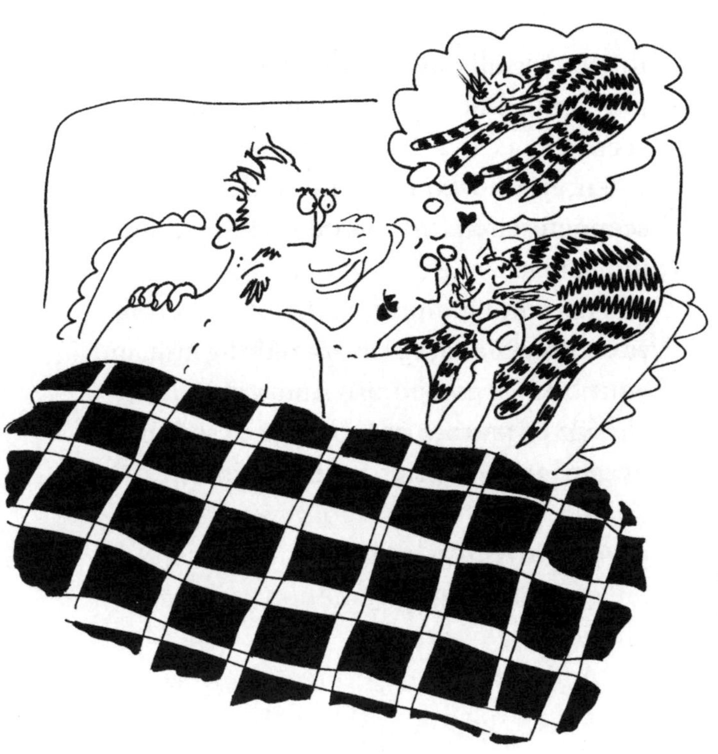

into it. We all have a tendency to be problem addicts – that's why we watch soap operas and disaster movies; but when the bad experiences in life start to seem more real than good ones, it's time to change.

If you've got into the habit of having sex with your mind on something else and your body switched off, it may not be a change of partner or a change of scene you need as much as a change of mind.

5. The Warm Up Exercise

The good news is that you do have some choice about how you experience your life in general and your sex life in particular.

This is what you do – and it's probably the easiest bit in the whole book. You don't need any help, any equipment or any mind-altering substances. Just your imagination. Find some private space and ten minutes peace and quiet to ask yourself these questions and *feel* the answers:

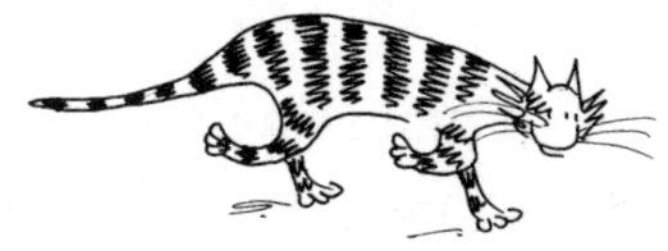

* What does good sex feel like? And where? The more places you get a tingle the better – after all, if you're only getting a twitch or two in the obvious places, that's a lot of wasted nerve-endings you could be putting to use.

* How long does it take?

* What does it smell like?

* What does it sound like?

* What does it taste like?

Keep practising this until you start to get some really good feelings in more than one or two locations and you know where and what they are.

HOW TO...

* This isn't a physical exercise, you don't have to *do* anything, except in your mind. And it's not a substitute for the real thing either, it's just a warm-up.

...DO IT

* Whatever you want, whether it's sex or world domination, you're more likely to succeed if you start by using your brain. The best sex definitely starts above the belt. Where it finishes is up to you.

Chapter Three

Natural Highs And Unnatural Lows

We learned about sex in biology lessons,
but as far as I'm concerned it's always been
pure chemistry.
HEDERA FOLEY

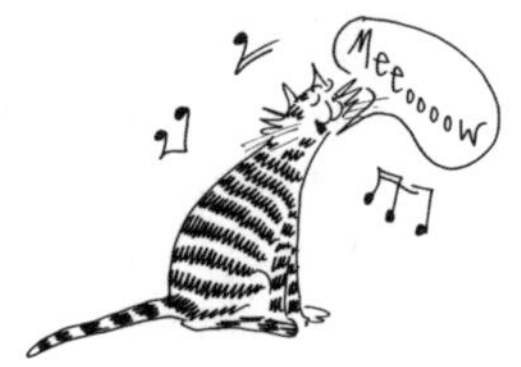

BENEFITS

* Good sex is easy when you know how to mix the right chemicals.

BONUS

* Adjusting your own hormones saves having to talk your doctor into giving you a prescription. It could also protect your health if you're tempted to get the juices flowing by illegal or unregulated methods.

Adjusting your own chemical balance isn't new. People did it long before Viagra. Almost any substance that was hard to get or weird to look at was used as an aphrodisiac at some time – although a lot of them did more for the supplier than the customer. Before there was lab testing, mixing sawdust and goose grease and selling it as unicorn horn was a major industry.

Of course a lot of this stuff worked quite well. If the aphrodisiac supplier was charismatic and convincing and the packaging looked good, it probably did the trick.

But now the pharmaceutical industry has taken the romance out of the aphrodisiac business by inventing synthetic hormones and drugs like Viagra which actually work. Although, if you prefer the natural approach you can still buy the powdered genitals of almost any endangered species from alternative suppliers – and they often come with a free crystal.

Natural Highs and Unnatural Lows

Drink, sir, ... it provokes the desire,
but it takes away the performance.
SHAKESPEARE

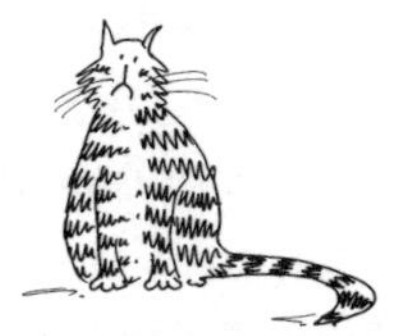

Then there are recreational drugs, which have been around for as long as recreational sex. We've got more choice than Shakespeare had – although alcohol is still the only legal one. Unfortunately brewers' droop doesn't only come with the beer – a number of currently fashionable substances also make you feel like you're having a better time than you really are.

Some of the legal 'feelgood' drugs have the same drawback – they do more for your mood than your performance. So think twice before you tell your doctor you're depressed about your love life – if she prescribes a designer drug you'll certainly feel happier, but you can forget about sex while you're taking the medicine. In fact, you *will* forget about sex while you're taking the medicine.

Porn is Viagra without the liver damage.
FAY WELDON

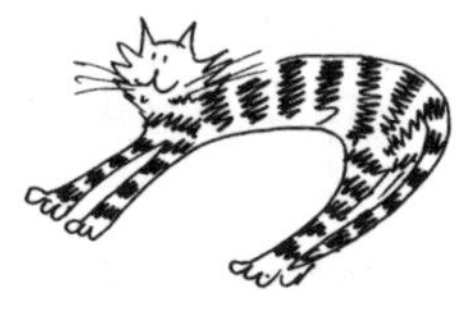

But if oysters and chocolate and ginkgo biloba don't guarantee multiple orgasms, if prescription drugs have side effects and recreational drugs aren't all they're cracked up to be, what are the alternatives? Pornography? Couples holidays? Ann Summers Parties? Therapy?

Even some of the more innocuous-sounding ideas should probably carry a health warning. As if sex itself wasn't wonderful and scary enough, it seems as though almost anything we do to improve it can be just as dangerous!

Take the 'try something different' advice in all the magazines. These articles used to be coyly called 'be more adventurous in the bedroom', but now it's more likely to be 'on the train' or 'under the restaurant table'.

I once worked in an office where coffee breaks were like True Confessions. The Head of IT was trying out every technique known to women's pages for putting the zing back into her sex life. Until one day she came into the office and announced she was thinking of divorce.

'We were fed up with pretending to be other people so we decided to be each other instead,' she said. 'Nigel admitted he'd always wanted to try on some of my clothes so we swapped – he's not that much taller than me. It was funny at first, he looked like Les Dawson in a skirt, but when I started putting his makeup on for him it all went wrong. I'd nearly finished doing his face and then I looked in the mirror and saw his Mum staring back at me. With a wig and mascara he looks exactly like her. I don't even want to think about sex with him now.'

If you want to quick fix your personal chemistry, it's faster and definitely safer to use your imagination than legal or illegal substances. But be prepared for unpredictable results. Still, that could be part of the fun, and fun is what it's all about.

1. The Magic Carpet Ride

A woman's idea of foreplay is a night at the opera, champagne, dinner and red roses but a man is turned on by six pints, a curry and Match of the Day.

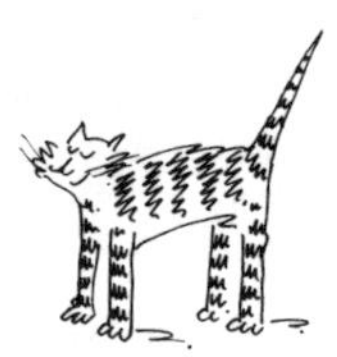

Anywhere is worth visiting if you travel by magic carpet. Whether it's a first date, a weekend in a long relationship or just solo, stopgap sex, the destination will be more exciting if you take the pretty route. The important things in life (sex, religion and politics) need rituals.

* A massage is a great pre-sex ritual. Anywhere or anything that makes your lover feel good will improve the end result for both of you. Take time to focus on your partner's body and your own feelings.

* A walk near trees or water puts you in touch with your natural energy (as opposed to walking down a busy street which simply stresses you).

* An exciting experience that gets your adrenaline going will generate some of the chemicals you need for sex. It could be a trip to the fair, a scary movie, a white water rafting trip, or even a parachute jump.

* A slow, elaborate meal has always been one of the greatest aphrodisiacs (and it doesn't have to be oysters). Lovingly prepared food is supposed to contain emotions as well as vitamins. It's worth a try.

Think about what's worked for *you* in the past and try some new ideas as well.

2. Setting Up For Success

If sex is more like scratching an itch than a cosmic explosion, try a different angle. Look beyond the experience itself and consider *where* you do it. If your car and your clothes reflect how you feel about yourself but your bedroom's uninspiring, what does that tell you?

* What do you associate with sex? Red velvet? A Moroccan harem? The back of the bike sheds? Go for a combination of sensual effect and memories of good times past.

* Do you like warm and cosy? Or dark and atmospheric? You might not want

dry ice or a roaring log fire on a nightly basis, but a touch of drama now and again could work wonders.

* Music is the food of love so turn on the stereo (not the radio – interruptions from car insurance ads ruin the mood). Don't make it too soothing and take into account the tastes of anyone else who's involved. Use music to keep the experience fresh – Bolero worked in the film, but playing it every night would probably be irritating.

* Smell is our most evocative sense, especially when it comes to primitive activities like sex and eating.

Chapter Three

Natural Highs and Unnatural Lows

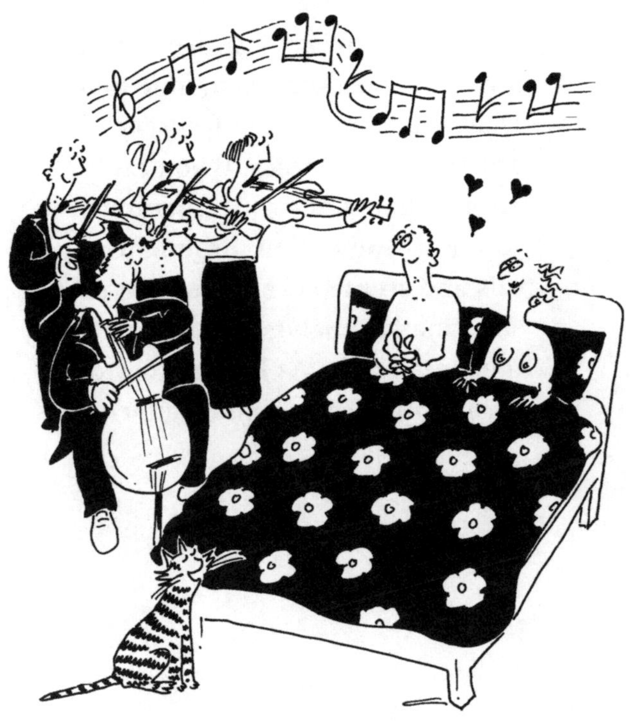

Experiment: instead of slapping on the latest perfume regardless of how it reacts on your skin, take time to test what smells make you feel sexy. There's lots of choice. If you can't afford Chanel or Cartier, perfume the room instead of you. Aromatherapy oils and scented candles are on the supermarket shelves and some of them are lovely. As long as they don't clash or trigger an asthma attack.

* And what about energy? Not your personal energy this time, but chi as in Feng Shui. Check that the room you use doesn't have any obviously dark or blocked corners and that there isn't a mirror or television facing the bed. See that the light flows gently and freely and lighting is warm and beautiful and subtle. Add some movement with plants, curtains or windchimes.

Have fun with rituals and settings. If you never gave it much thought before, a few simple changes could make a lot of difference.

HOW TO...

* Take time to plan the next time you have sex. Imagine it's the first time, the time of your life.

* Experiment with different ideas and activities – one at a time if you don't want to burn out or frighten your partner.

...DO IT

* Don't put off having sex 'til you've redecorated your house or hired a string quartet. Make some simple changes and get started.

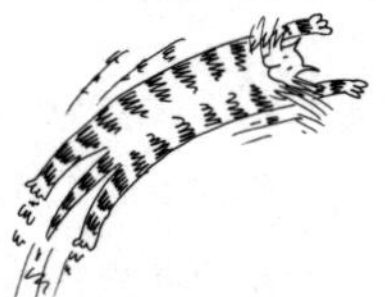

Chapter Four

Relax, Don't Do It

Sex is really all in the mind, not the body.
VIRGINIA IRONSIDE

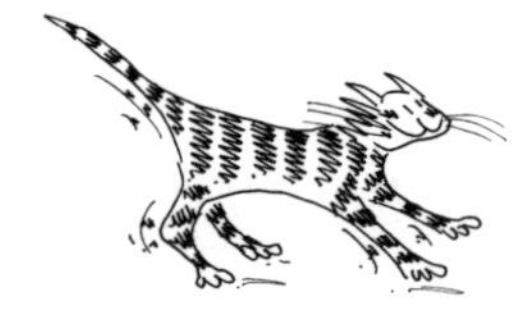

BENEFITS

* Giving yourself permission not to have sex unless you really want it gives you the possibility of enjoying it again.

* Life is less stressful when you're living your own agenda rather than somebody else's.

BONUS

* Freeing yourself from compulsory sex for a while may put the rest of your life into perspective as well.

Now we can protect ourselves from disease and pregnancy, there's no need for a social taboo on sex. This takes away some of the compulsion to do it of course. Forbidden things are always more desirable.

If aliens decided to check us out before bothering to invade, they could start in any corner shop and browse through what we read. Glancing through popular magazines makes it obvious that our main preoccupations are dieting, shopping and sex.

Sex has never been top of those must-haves. Currently in women's magazines it takes second place to slimming and shopping. And the sex articles that aren't just soft porn are becoming more like extracts from a graphic self-help manual. There's a last-ditch-desperate feel to some of them that makes you feel you ought to be making more effort.

In fact, the trouble with sex nowadays is that there are far too many oughts and shoulds about it. It was probably more fun when there were more ought nots and should nots. The Victorians thought sex was such a powerful force that they put frills on the furniture as well as the women to stop lewd thoughts derailing polite conversation. If the sight of an uncovered table leg was considered likely to throw male dinner guests into fits of lust nowadays, maybe they wouldn't need Viagra.

Right now, if you aren't doing it as often as James Bond, you'd better keep quiet. It's just not on to admit that sex isn't top of your daily agenda, especially if you're fashionable and famous – or would like to be. Fading media stars often use sex to fuel a comeback, either by acquiring a glitzy, young partner, or by writing a book about how raunchy their life has been. A glamorous wedding invitation arrived recently – triple layer gauze and parchment with silver ribbon. I wasn't surprised because I knew my friend's daughter was engaged, but then I looked again. It wasn't Jenny's daughter who was getting married, it was Jenny herself. 'But she's only just divorced,' I thought. Then I noticed that she was remarrying her ex-husband, so I grabbed the phone.

'All our friends were separating,' she said, 'and they kept telling us how exciting it was to be screwing around again, so we thought we'd give it a go. We both felt we ought to get out and see a bit of life before we're too old.'

'So what happened?' I asked her.

'Well, we missed each other so we thought we'd put some excitement back into things by remarrying. Everybody thinks it's very romantic and completely mad so it's almost as good as having an unsuitable affair. All the benefits with none of the risk.'

Later, over dinner, I asked her ex-husband/fiancé for his view of things. 'Expensive,' he said, 'but better than living on my own and less trouble than starting from scratch. I can't be bothered to go out looking for sex when I can get it at home and watch Match of the Day as well.'

Chapter Four

Relax, Don't Do It

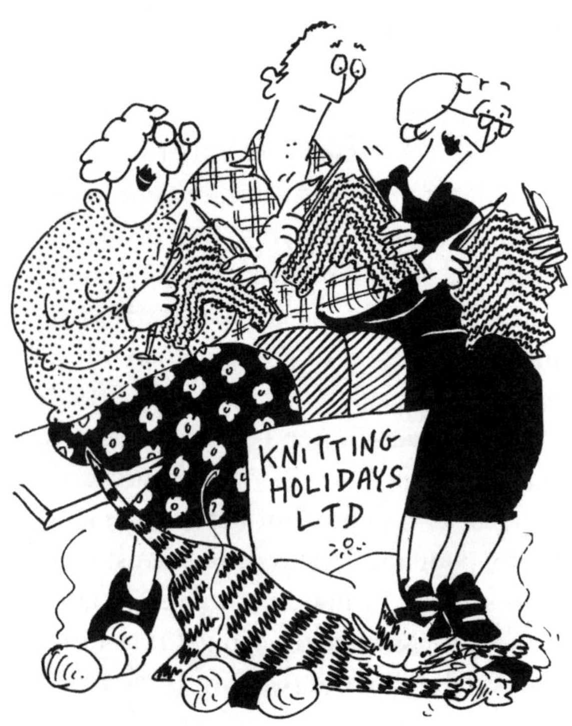

1. Take Time Out

If you really want more sex, or you just want to think about sex more often, why not take time out? Instead of going on a sex, sun and sand holiday, do something different.

* Go on a retreat for a week and don't think about sex.

* Take a special interest holiday doing something you already enjoy or want to learn about (not sex). Make it something that's unlikely to include any attractive people. You could lie about your age (if you're under 50) and join a Saga gardening tour, but there are plenty of painting, writing,

welding and astronomy courses in nice parts of the world. Lose yourself in an activity where you aren't under pressure to pull.

* If neither of these options are drastic enough and you really want to get sex into perspective, sign up for a long-distance sailing race or an Arctic trek.

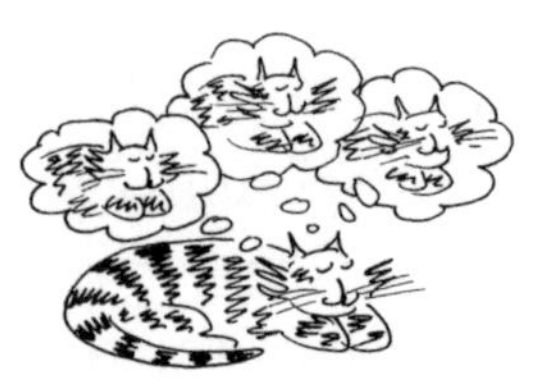

2. Take Time

If you have a regular partner and you both agree that sex is so dire you need outside help, a currently popular therapy is not doing it at all for a while, followed by a period of not doing it all. There are many different versions of this from DIY (or rather don't) tantric sex to the Relate Sensate Focus Programme.

It's like suddenly having rules again – only this time you, your partner and your therapist make them up. But, you still have to stick to them – otherwise it don't work.

* *Week One.* Spend half an hour with your partner every day, holding hands and talking. Eye contact is important. For the rest of the time you're allowed to share everything but sex, especially mealtimes if you don't normally eat together.

* *Week Two.* Take an hour a day for at least five days a week and go to bed with your partner. You are allowed to touch and talk – but no sex.

* *Week Three.* Again, spend that hour a day in bed, but this time focus on another activity such as listening to music or playing cards. Touching and talking is allowed, but no sex or TV.

* ***Week Four.*** Give each other a massage for five days out of seven.

Day One	hands
Day Two	neck and head
Day Three	back
Day Four	feet
Day Five	all over

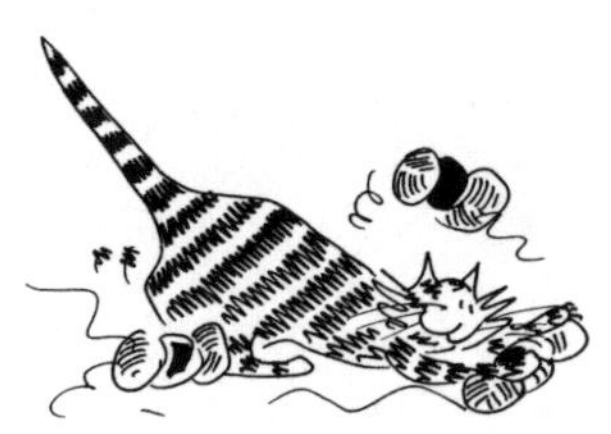

Days One to Four must be done in silence but on Day Five give feedback to your partner about what feels good and what you would like them to do for you.

There are a thousand different versions of this and the rules will evolve depending on how quickly the process is working for you.

3. Playtime

Typically, when people fall in love and sex is good, they are very playful. A lot of time is spent being pretty childish. Look at the language in the personal columns on Valentine's Day.

If you want to have good sex with someone, take time out first and do something else that's fun and puts you into a relaxed or irresponsible frame of mind.

* A summertime trip to the seaside at dawn, arriving for breakfast and leaving before lunch. You could go home then and catch up on some sleep.

* Hire a rowing boat and spend an afternoon on the river.

* Challenge your partner to a round of crazy golf or a game of Scrabble.

* Take a trip to the fair and go on some of the scary rides (anything that feels a little dangerous can also make you feel sexy – see Chapter Three).

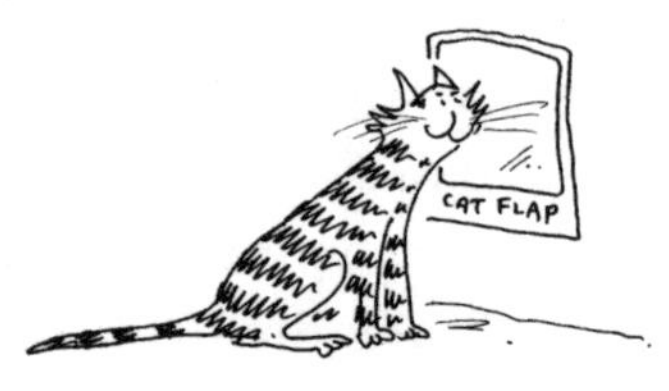

HOW TO...

* Exercise Two is for long-term relationships – talk it through with your partner first.
* Exercises One and Three only work if you have fun doing them. If they add to your *'must, should and ought'* list, don't bother.

...DO IT

* If you've spent too much time trying too hard to have good sex, you deserve some time off. Give yourself space to get your breath and your appetite back.

Chapter Five

Me First?

Sex is a gift you allow yourself to have – like happiness – if you feel you deserve it.
KATE STACEY

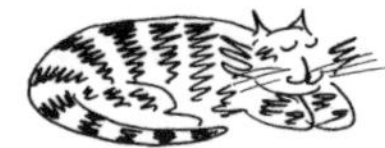

BENEFITS

* Caring for yourself gives you the confidence to choose a better sex life.

* Looking good conveys the message that you enjoy your body and cherish it – and that you expect others to do the same.

BONUS

* Your appearance affects the way other people treat you, so look after yourself. Other people will treat you better and then you will feel more confident.

We all walk around wearing invisible designer labels and price tags which most other human beings can clearly read. If your label says: *'Human football, six careless owners. Going cheap'*, guess what sort of attention you are going to attract? The trouble is, you can't arbitrarily repackage yourself. It's not that easy. If you don't *believe* the new label you try to stick on yourself, the glue won't work.

People who like themselves hang out with other people who like them. People who don't like themselves will look for the kind of company that confirms their self-image.

People who like themselves get the best things in life. Sex included.

Thirty-five years ago, a new girl joined our girl's school sixth form. Her parents were Venezuelan and she'd travelled the world. We were knocked out by how exotic she was although we didn't like her much because she was different. However, we were curious, so every day she'd fill us in on the graphic details of her night before and we were impressed.

We thought she was probably showing off – but we weren't sure. Then she suddenly left. The teachers didn't deny the pregnancy rumours though the official notice said 'family relocation'.

Ten years later, I saw her on television – a journalist in a war-torn area of the world, looking glamorous in camouflage and bravely holding up a microphone under fire.

Twenty years later I met her at a school reunion. By this time she was famous enough to be guest of honour and gave a very entertaining keynote speech. Afterwards, we were all desperate to meet her – not that we gave a damn about her exciting life, there was only one thing we wanted to know. 'Did you really have a baby?'

'Of course', she said. 'I wanted an abortion, but my family wouldn't allow it and I'm glad of that now. I get on well with my son – he wants to be a journalist.'

'Are you married?' we asked, 'or have you still got as many boyfriends?'

She started to laugh. 'I haven't got time. I used to talk about sex a lot because it was the only way I could get your attention. I don't need it now – I have a great life and everybody knows who I am.'

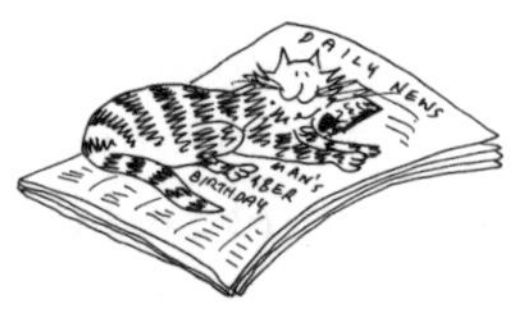

Sex is never going to be a great experience if it's just a way of getting attention or proving to yourself that you're attractive. Good sex happens to people who think they deserve it. So what's the Quick Fix route to an orgasmic sense of self-worth? You don't need to be famous. The only person you need to impress is you.

1. Affirmations

Is sex dirty?
Only if it's done right.
WOODY ALLEN

The power of regular affirmations is something we all know about but are usually too embarrassed to do. But affirmations aren't as embarrassing as good sex ought to be, so have another go:

* Keep it short and in the present tense: *'I am sexy'*.

* Repeat it twenty times a day and before you go to sleep.

* Write it on your shaving mirror, on the back of your wardrobe door and in your underwear drawers.

* If you're not self-conscious stick it on the fridge and the inside the front door as well. Don't put it on the outside of the front door.

If it still doesn't feel convincing or dynamic enough, try singing it. You can get an idea to loop round your brain much more easily if it's set to music. Almost anything by Tom Jones will do but if you really can't identify with him, pick yourself another role model with appropriate lyrics.

2. Maintenance

It's a status symbol for a woman to be high maintenance these days and men are catching up fast. But there are still too many men (and women) who look after their cars much more lovingly than they care for themselves. A French friend of mine couldn't understand why all the men in our street were cleaning their cars on a Sunday morning. 'Why aren't they in bed having a good time?' she said, 'or getting over the good time they had last night? Don't you have carwashes here?'

- Cars are a sex symbol of course, but why not skip the symbolism and go for the real thing. Springclean your personal bodywork and see if anyone's impressed. *You'll* feel better in it even if nobody else notices.

- Look after your hair and your skin. Whether you're male or female, these are the basics and it's not about fashion or image – just about valuing yourself.

- Review your clothes. Do they look and feel good to you? If you met yourself in a singles bar would you want to take yourself home?

Being high maintenance has different meanings for different people, so before you move to the next exercise, take a moment to check out what it means to you. Having highlights in your hair because it makes you feel good is not the same as having it done because you're afraid people might reject grey old you. If you've got any doubts about your motivation, have your hair done anyway but repeat the mantra *'because I'm worth it'* while you're in the stylist's chair.

Chapter Five

Me First?

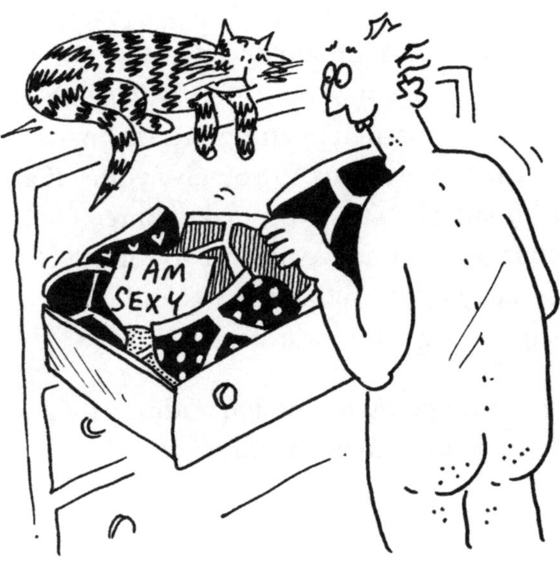

3. Be Your Own Agent

Imagine you're a famous sex symbol with an image to maintain and that you are your own agent. Your career is flagging and you just aren't getting the sexy parts in the hottest films so you give yourself an ultimatum. Either you make some changes or you give up and go for the comedy roles, character parts and supporting actor awards.

* Am I going to enough auditions – am I serious about being sexy?

* How am I saying my lines? Do I sound like a dental drill? (if you aren't sure, record yourself and listen to the playback). If you can't afford a voice coach just slow down and lower your pitch.

* Do I look the part I want to play?

4. Treat Yourself

Fit as much sensual pleasure into your life as you can stand. Good sex is about being in touch with your physical needs.

* Take a few minutes longer over your baths or showers and use scented oils and body lotion.

* Every day prepare and eat something simple but delicious without doing something else at the same time. It could be a banana sandwich or a bowl of cereal, but make sure you are really hungry and linger over the tastes and textures.

* As often as you can afford the time and money, treat yourself to the kind of saunas, massages and beauty treatments you enjoy.

Avoid easy escape routes (like watching TV) and install more good feelings into your life. Turn up the pleasure instead of numbing the pain.

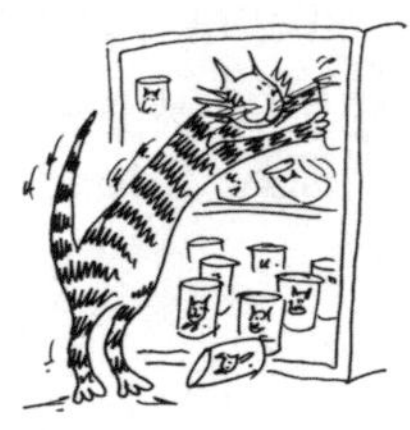

HOW TO…

* Everything you do must make you *feel* good as well as look good. If it doesn't tickle your erogenous zones as well as your self-esteem, don't do it. Take pleasure in your own appearance.

…DO IT

* Make sensual treats a routine. If you haven't got time to do these little things for yourself right now, how will you fit regular sex into your busy schedule anyway?

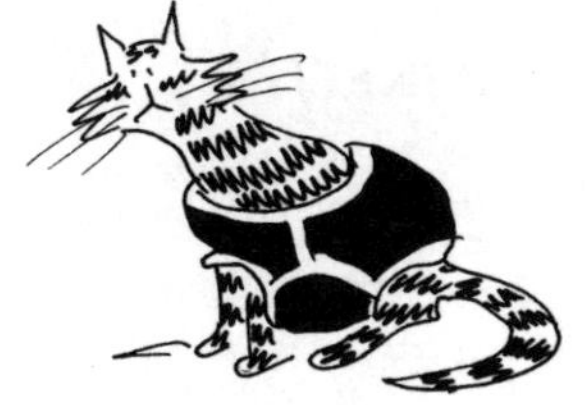

Chapter Six

Fit?

You'd better shape up...
SATURDAY NIGHT FEVER

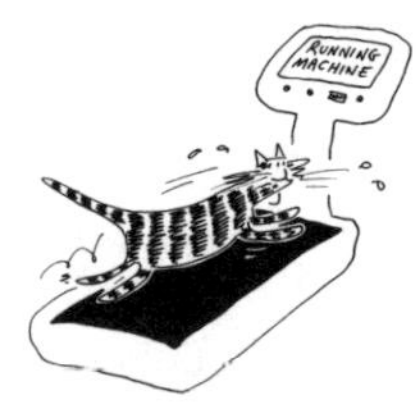

BENEFITS

* People who are in good shape have more choices when it comes to sex.

* Sex is better when you're fit enough to keep it up for longer.

BONUS

* If you start working out in the hope of improving your sex life you'll find yourself feeling healthier all round. So you could be extending your sex life as well as upgrading it.

* Joining any kind of club that involves exercise, whether it's a rowing club, a squash club or the local gym, is a great way to meet fit potential partners.

Doris, my elderly neighbour, asked me the title of the book I was writing. '*Quick Fix Your Sex Life*,' I said, feeling embarrassed. 'You had to be very fit to have sex when I was a girl,' said Doris.

When I asked her what she meant, she explained 'well, we only had bicycles because it was during the war, and we couldn't do it at home.'

Petrol rationing aside, we are genetically programmed to look for partners who are healthy enough to produce the next generation. For thousands of years, the strongest men attracted the most fertile-looking women and the women with the biggest hips and boobs and smallest waists attracted the most powerful men. Now that we have IVF and social services, physical strength isn't so important for childrearing. But it's essential for recreational sex. If your blood pressure is low, your muscle tone is high and you've got stamina, sex is going to be better than if you get breathless climbing the bedroom stairs.

I had lunch recently with two friends I hadn't seen for ages. One of them was newly married and the other newly divorced and it sounded like the two emotional agendas were incompatible. I wasn't expecting it to be fun.

Looking around the restaurant, I couldn't see either of them. Then I noticed them waving at me from a corner.

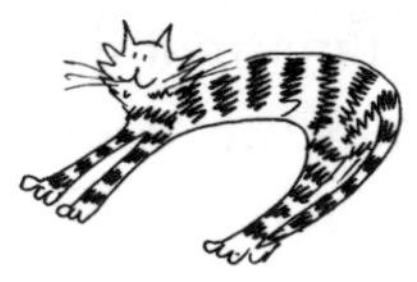

They both looked terrible. And Jane who had just got married looked even rougher than Beth who was divorced. 'You didn't recognise us, did you?' they said accusingly. I made an excuse about not having my glasses.

'You don't have to be polite,' said Beth. 'I know I look like nothing on earth, but what's the point? It's just me and the kids and by the time they're old enough for me to go out again, I'll be past caring about having a sex life.' Then she challenged Jane: 'So what's your excuse? You've only been married six months – you aren't pregnant, are you?'

Jane was indignant. 'No I'm not. Being married means that you can be yourself. You don't have to pretend anymore.'

'You mean you can't be bothered to go to the gym anymore', said Beth, 'and now you've got him you don't think you have to make an effort. I fell into that trap – next thing you know he'll be walking out with a size eight in high heels.'

It's no good blaming your sluggish sex life on the fact that your partner looks like one of the Slobs. Trying to turn someone else into a sex god or goddess amounts to nagging, not loving care. You only get results by investing that time and attention in yourself. Lead by example.

And if your chosen partner doesn't follow that example, you have a choice. A tough one, admittedly, but it's still a choice. After all, what does it say about you if the person you're having sex with has let themselves go?

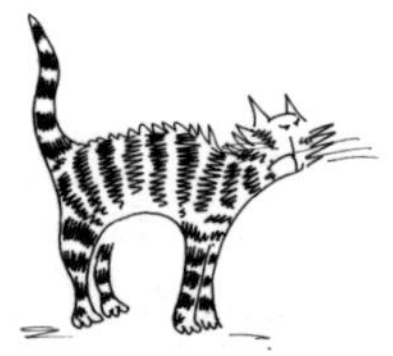

1. Join a gym

Regular articles in women's (and men's) magazines with titles like *Shag Yourself Thin*, and *Horizontal Jogging*, suggest sex is a good way to keep fit. But they don't give facts and figures. Laboratory studies of sexual activity don't usually measure the number of calories burned during an average session. And what's an average session anyway?

The safest bet is to play it safe and assume you're going to have to get fit in order to get more sex, rather than assuming that more sex will keep you fit.

You can work out at home, but if you're starting from scratch it's better to go to a health club and get a programme designed for you by a personal trainer. If you tell her what you're training for, she might even come up with some helpful suggestions!

* Build up some muscle. There's nothing more humiliating than trying an adventurous new position and finding your biceps aren't up to it. Or putting your back out (this is quite common apparently).

* Stamina is important, so jog or cycle or go to aerobics classes. This kind of exercise makes you look good *and* feel good. It releases endorphins into your bloodstream making you calmer and

Chapter Six

Fit?

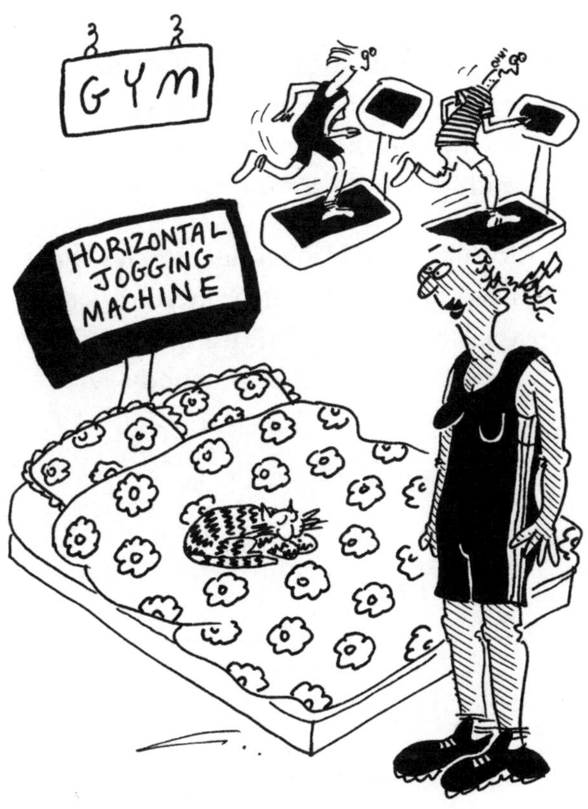

more optimistic – which will make you more fun to be with as well as giving you the confidence to go out and look for a good time.

* It's not just the obvious muscles that need exercise. Women often neglect their pelvic floor but learning to flex it for fun could make somebody very happy.

2. Stay in shape

Sex symbols tend not to be stick thin; heroin chic may be fashionable but it isn't sexy. But fat isn't sexy either. Being built for comfort rather than speed is all very well, but it's difficult to have an active sex life when just being active is difficult enough.

* Taking enough exercise is more important than watching what you eat if you want to stay slim.

* Of course eating habits do make some difference. If you want to be in better shape for better sex, learn to eat when you're hungry and stop when you're full. It's as simple as that. Calorie

counting doesn't work – in fact it's more likely to make you obsessed with what you can't eat. Maybe you could try being obsessional about sex instead – it's not as fattening.

* The third factor in staying slim and sexy is to eat healthy food. Your sex life will suffer if you don't have all the nutrients you need, but get them from a varied diet rather than by loading up with pills. After all, a bowl of fruit is more fun to share than a bottle of trace mineral capsules.

HOW TO...

* Once you start exercising, you'll feel the difference fast. Start gently and build up.

* Make it something you enjoy, if it's fun, you'll keep it up. Physical pleasure is a good habit to get into.

...DO IT

* Keeping fit and eating well could become a way of life. Something you deserve and take for granted, instead of a stop/start health and fitness pattern that depends on the state of your relationships.

Chapter Seven

Pressing the Right Buttons

I don't want to talk about my sex life
– it's a bit messy at the moment. And that's exactly how I like it!
DELANEY HOUSTON III

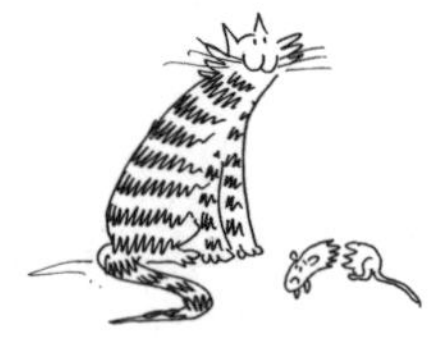

BENEFITS

* When you take a reality check on your sex life you can start to make the changes you want but you can't put right problems you don't know about.

BONUS

* Insights into what makes sex work for you, or against you, will give you a better perspective on other important bits of your life as well.

Apparently we are 80% emotionally programmed at eight years old. So whatever messages about sex we got at that age, and younger, could still be affecting us now. You may not remember what specific bits of bad advice you were given – but that won't stop you acting on them.

Pressing the Right Buttons

My best friend's father bred rabbits and one day after school he sent Susan and me to borrow a couple of male rabbits from his friend – to expand the gene pool I suppose. Or maybe his current rabbits had complained that they were bored with each other.

We carried one basket each and knocked at his friend's door. 'My Dad is borrowing Ernie's prize shaggers,' said Susan, innocently.

Ernie's wife looked disapproving. She grabbed both the baskets and told us to wait. 'Can't we have a look at all your other rabbits?' we asked.

'No you can't. They might be – you know ...'

'Shagging?' we said hopefully.

Chapter Seven
Pressing the Right Buttons

By the time we got back to Susan's house with the two rabbits, the phone lines had been buzzing and we were in trouble. 'What did you have to let me down like that for?' said her Dad.

'Like what?' we said. 'She wouldn't even let us see Ernie's rabbits in case they were ... you know...' Before we'd have said it without thinking. But in the space of an hour, we'd learned that something we'd always taken for granted (with rabbits at least) was actually pretty controversial and that different people had different rules about what was OK and what wasn't.

1. Finding the Bugs

Which of these words describes your sex life right now (choose at least three):

Active
Boring
Childish
Comforting
Dangerous
Depressing
Detached
Dirty
Disinterested
Disassociated
Dull
Dutiful
Ecstatic
Emotional
Excessive
Exotic
Expensive
Forbidden
Frantic
Frustrating
Funny
Furtive
Fussy
Glamorous
Guilty
Happy
Hard work
Hysterical

Immature
Inactive
Inadequate
Inconvenient
Inevitable
Interesting
Longing
Loving
Mechanical
Messy
Middle aged
Mundane
Normal
Obligatory
Ordinary
Passionate
Passive
Physical
Pornographic
Repressed
Romantic
Sad
Sinful
Sordid
Steady
Strenuous
Stressful
Tiring
Unavoidable
Unimportant
Violent
Weird
Wild
Wonderful

Now take the words you chose and divide them into positive and negative. Make sure that you know what is positive and what is negative for you. For example, *'dangerous'* might be a positive description for some people but not for others and so might *'weird'* or *'funny'*. It's what it means to you that matters.

Positive **Negative**

Which column is the longest?
Does anything surprise you?
Does it tell you anything you didn't know?

Chapter Seven

Pressing the Right Buttons

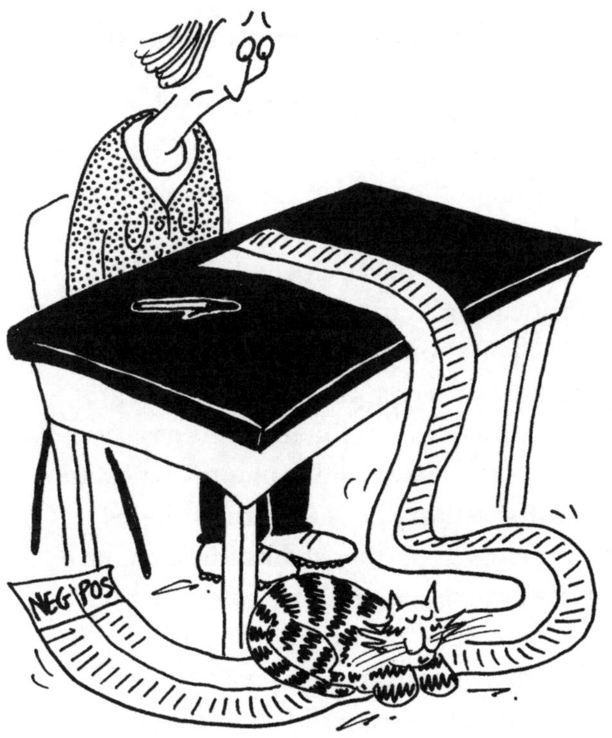

2. De-bugging the programme

You've just run a double-check on your feelings about sex, which has probably confirmed the glitches you already knew about. But just take a moment to make sure that you haven't been hijacked by political correctness. Are you sure that what you thought was a problem isn't really your secret preference? After all, if you want your sex life to be hysterical and immature, or sad and romantic, who's to say it shouldn't be? Of course it helps if your chosen partner shares the same taste in sex as you do, and if they don't, you're going to have to change your mind or change your partner. Or give up sex.

When you're confident that you know

what's good for you and what isn't, the next step is to take a look at *where* your negative messages about sex are coming from. Because then you can find the Off switch. Or at least turn the volume down.

It's amazing how often we mismanage important areas of our life simply because we are living by somebody else's rules, old beliefs that just aren't relevant to us any more (if they ever were) and outdated information. Taking a backward glance to where some of this negative stuff came from often makes us realise that we can get rid of it for good. And you don't have to go through five years of psychoanalysis to do it – you can run a 'quick and dirty' right now and get it out into the light of day.

If you have a special partner, do this exercise together. That way you can check each other's programmes for compatibility. There's a health warning on this though: if you have any traumatic issues on the subject of childhood and sex, put this book down immediately and get some help with defusing them. You don't have to live with those problems – but you aren't going to solve them by reading a book. There is some brilliant expert advice available, so do some research and find the right person to help you de-bug.

If you're ready to go ahead, get together with your partner or your best buddy and see if you can entertain each other with the answers to the next few questions. You can do it alone if you prefer – but that might say something about your sex life too. There's just one rule: each story you tell must raise a smile. Even if it wasn't funny at the time, lighten it up as you re-tell it.

* When was the first time you remember being aware of sex?
* Who told you the facts of life – or did you always know?
* Can you recall an embarrassing sex-related family incident?
* When did you realise your parents – or any other adults – had a sexual relationship?

3. Cleaning Up The Drive

Next check for any other relevant patterns and where they might be. Start whenever your sex life did. For example:

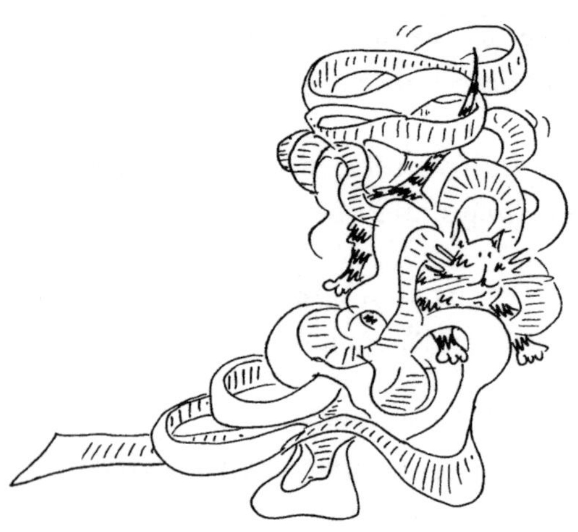

TIME	**SCORE 1–10** *1 = no sex* *10 = ecstatic*	**RELEVANT FACTORS**
1994-97	*8*	*Went to college – living away from home for the first time*
1997	*9*	*Exciting new job, travelling a lot, long distance relationship with girl in New York*
1998-9	*1*	*Girlfriend gets pregnant by somebody else. Break off relationship*
2000	*3*	*Lose job and live with parents again. Start relationship with girl next door*

Now that you have assembled a few more bits of the jigsaw that makes up your sex life, what could you consciously change that would make a difference – an improvement – in the future? However bad things are, don't be defeated before you start by thinking you have to change everything. Just one change will domino-effect lots of others.

* What beliefs have been running my sex life up to now? What do I think sex is for? Fun? Having children? Cementing relationships? Keeping the peace? Proving I'm lovable? Do I want to keep my current beliefs, or could I ditch some of them?

* Am I confident about my own sexual preferences and do I live my life accordingly?

* What has affected my sex life, now or in the past? Techniques, types of relationship, life factors (like a fulfilling job), or lifestyle patterns (like being financially independent).

* What stops me from using those techniques again, or having those relationships or that lifestyle which made me happy in the past?

4. Testing the programme

Finally, ask yourself:

* What steps am I going to take to make positive changes starting from now?
* When am I going to start?

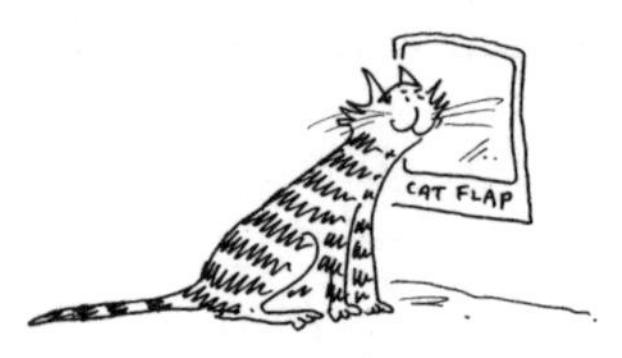

HOW TO...

* Don't linger over the analysis, get through that bit as fast as you can and decide to change. If you spend too much time on the original problems you might even reinforce those outdated beliefs and make the traumas seem more powerful than they really were.

...DO IT

* Start immediately. Identify something in your life that you will change tomorrow (or today) and make a difference. It could be starting a relationship – or finishing an old one. Or embracing a whole new lifestyle.

Chapter Eight

GSOH

(Sex) was the most fun I ever had without laughing.
WOODY ALLEN

BENEFITS

* If you ask enough questions, one of the answers you get is bound to be right.

* Asking questions helps define the difference between what you really want and what you think you ought to have.

BONUS

* Figuring out the true cost of your ideal sex life means that you've already taken the first step towards getting it.

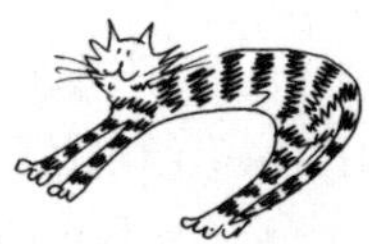

It's time to ask again the question in Chapter One: do you know exactly what sort of sex life you want and how it would feel if you got it?

I was giving a talk on contraception to a girls' school sixth form some years ago and thought I'd start with the basics. On the board I wrote 'What's a normal sex life?'

One of the girls raised her hand. 'I don't want a normal sex life,' she said 'I want an amazing, earth-shattering, ten-orgasm-a-night sort of sex life.'

'What's an orgasm?' asked the girl sitting behind her.

It's easy to want it all when you've no idea what it's all about. But if you're going to get something worth having, the first step is to define it in detail. Otherwise you're likely to get stuck with the first option (or person) that comes your way and offers you heaven on a plate. Or at least a quickie after dinner. If you define what you want, you won't get distracted so easily and the wrong sort of sex life can be very distracting indeed.

Chapter Eight

GSOH

zzZ
ORGASM GOAL SETTING
WEEK 1
10
K 2
15
K 3
20
K 4
30
WEEK 5
45
WEEK 6
60
K 7
80
100

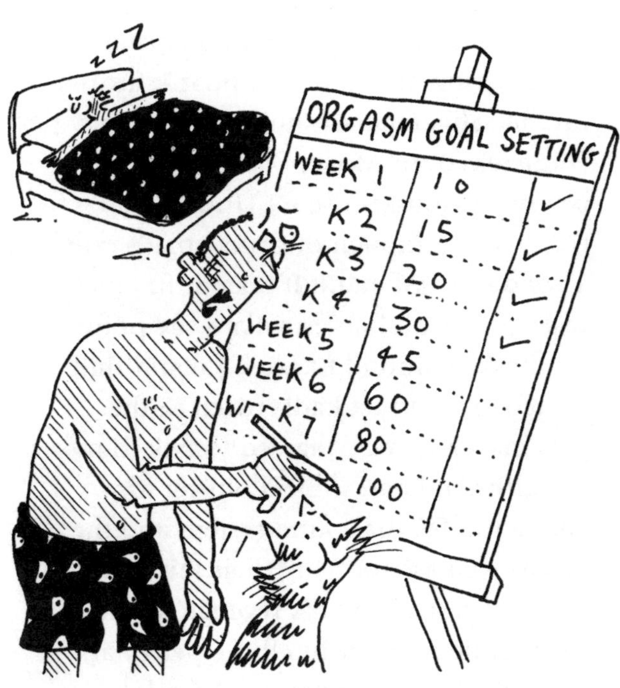

Chapter Eight

GSOH

Have you noticed the personal columns in magazines and newspapers? Considering how different people are, why do they all sound so similar in the *Find A Partner* section? Most people don't get beyond a Good Sense Of Humour (GSOH) – although of course that's quite a good start. After all, if it's not fun and you don't want babies, what's the point?

I asked around to see if I could find somebody who had advertised in the personals and a guy agreed to talk to me. His girlfriend had walked out on him, taking the TV, the sound system and the cats as well as emptying their joint bank account, so he took his revenge by posting her mobile number in all the personal columns. 'What did you put?' I asked

'Bear in mind' he said, 'that a lot of people answering those ads are looking for free sex, not real relationships. If you phrase it carefully you can screen out the genuine punters altogether.' He opened the magazine and pointed: *lively blonde seeks someone to get addicted to*. 'That means: *I'm trying to give up the other substances and I need a substitute.* And look at this: *loves cosy evenings in*, that probably means *I'm too weird to have a social life*.'

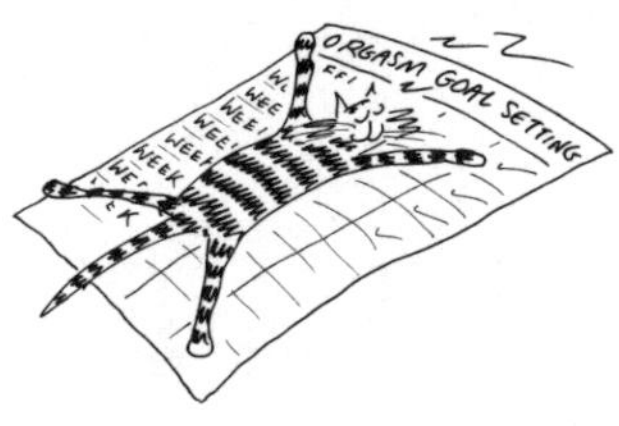

Then he produced his own ad, with his ex-girlfriend's phone number at the end. *Striking, independent brunette needs excitement. I'm not into wealth and status or even looks. I just want to get to know you for yourself.*

'What do you think?' he said triumphantly, 'that should have netted a pretty good selection of no-hopers, S&M merchants and con artists.'

1. For Sale

Imagine you're selling your current sex life in the used column of the Sunday paper. How would you describe it? And what price would you ask?

How about: *'Comfortable sex life, with interesting features. Needs constant attention due to age and doesn't do long distances. Bodywork sound but needs touching up. Not as exciting as it used to be, but very regular – minimum fortnightly. Good basic working order. Price: annual income of £30,000 plus cups of tea in bed and two holidays a year.'*

Or would that be overselling it?

2. Wanted

Now write the ad for your future sex life. The one you really want. What would you be willing to pay for that? What would you actually go without to have sex like you have in your dreams? After all, a lot of people (especially when they reach a certain point in middle age) do give up their homes and families, their jobs and their lifestyles just so they can recapture the sexual excitement of their teens. Or perhaps the dream of sex they never had.

So what do you want?

'Excitement, new places, new person / people, new positions, a loving relationship, glamour, romance, eternal youth?'

And what are you willing to pay? Your current sex life is the minimum down payment, but you may have to top it up.

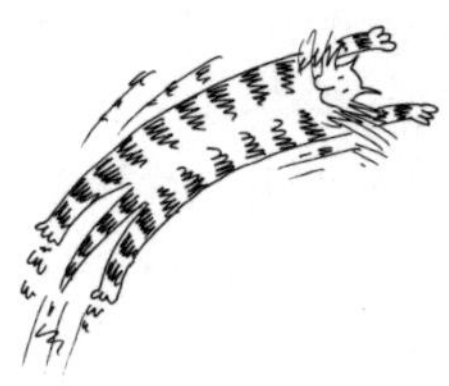

3. Part Exchange

If you can't put a price on what you want, maybe you could go for an exchange. Because, if your sex life is currently not great, it might be because you are doing something else.

Sex is such a basic instinct that if you aren't doing it, the hole may get filled by another activity. And sometimes that works really well – after all, if you can channel your sexual energy into your work or your art or your politics, just think how dynamic you could be. Sadly, the mundane displacement activities that most of us resort to when we aren't getting enough sex have more negative side effects. Overeating, for example, which is one of the more popular sex substitutes, makes you fat. And the fatter you get, the less attractive you are and the more difficult it is to have sex ... But in spite of that, a chocolate mousse is an orgasmic experience for an awful lot of people.

So think about that chocolate mousse, or glass of wine, or cigarette, or that frenetic work pattern. What do you get out of those activities that you could also get out of sex? Given that safe sex is better for our health than most of the alternatives, what's stopping you from going back to the real thing?

4. The Price of Reality

If you were to write the story of your perfect holiday romance or sexual experience – how would it read? Take the time now to jot down a synopsis and a bit of detail. Is it a Barbara Cartland? Something off the top shelf? Or even more extreme than that? Would Smiths actually sell it? Could you be arrested if it was discovered on your laptop?

5. Cybersex

And speaking of laptops – do you need real sex at all? A lot of people settle for the fantasy version either on video or the internet. There are lots of benefits: it's cheap, the timing is flexible, there are limitless possibilities and you don't have to make any effort at all. And of course, it really is the safest sex.

6. The Ultimate Question

Now that you've had time to consider, are you willing, or able, to meet the cost of the sex life you really want?

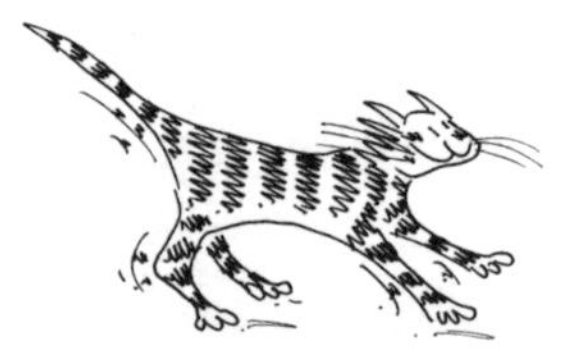

HOW TO...

* Write your ad and your story and ask yourself, first, if it's really what you want and, secondly, how much you are willing to pay.

...DO IT

* When you've made your choice, make your first downpayment. What's it going to be? Will you sacrifice your nights in front of the TV to get out and meet new people? Could you lose that weight you promised yourself so that you'll have the confidence to take your clothes off in front of someone?

Chapter Nine

Income-patibility

Never, ever, no matter what else you do in your whole life, never sleep with anyone whose troubles are worse than your own.

NELSON ALGREN

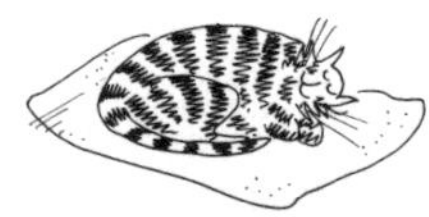

BENEFITS

* The best sex happens when you empty your mind and concentrate on your body. Here are some ways to clear the mental clutter so you can get on with whatever you want to do.

BONUS

* The ideas in this chapter give you a framework for carefree sex – and might save you time and alimony.

This chapter only applies if your sex life involves co-operation from another human being. If not, you could reconsider the cybersex option. Or go for a displacement activity and become a workaholic, or a football fan or a campaigner for lost causes.

But if you want real sex with real people regardless of the mess, the heartache and the paperwork, there are a few things you can do to protect yourself from the fallout.

Chapter Nine

Income-patibility

They divorced because he didn't have an income and she wasn't pattable.

MUSIC HALL JOKE

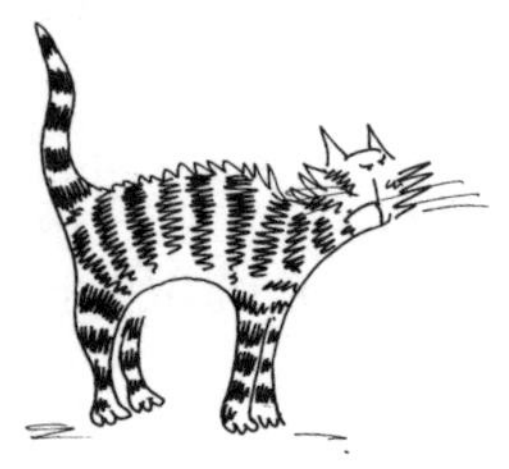

OK, it's terrible – but not sexist. You can substitute he for she and vice versa – or put together any combination you like. But when it comes to the crunch, any sex-based relationship needs two things, attraction and income. So a deal has to be put together. It may be a short-term deal or a long-term one, but some sort of deal there has to be – even if it's only an agreement about time and place.

There's no free lunch – and no free sex. It always costs something, even if it's only a glass of wine, a massage, or some of your precious time. So, if you want a good deal, you'd better make up your mind exactly what you want and what it's worth. After all, you get what you pay for.

Joe was one of the handsomest men I ever met, and one of the most insecure. A male model who supplemented his income by working for an escort agency, he was a charming, well-read and attentive companion. His friends – male and female – all adored him, but our friendship wasn't enough. We weren't surprised when he started a relationship with one of his clients – a city accountant he escorted to company functions. She was ten years older and highly successful.

At the engagement party I noticed that her house was perfect. Even the Siamese cat was a tasteful shade of beige to match the rugs and Joe looked more like the accessory of the moment than man of the house.

Two months later, they were married, and two years later, when their baby was a year old, they divorced. Joe came round to see me with his little boy. 'I'll have to get a job,' he said, gloomily, 'and that means I can't look after him any more. All she wanted was a baby, she didn't really want me.'

Since I'd drawn that conclusion anyway, there wasn't much I could say. 'What about the divorce settlement?' I asked.

'It only covers the kid,' he said. 'She did a pre-nuptial agreement. I didn't bother to read it at the time, but I have now. It runs to fifty pages and she even listed her CDs. I should have seen it coming and stuck with casual sex.'

1. Working out a deal

Sex used to be just one factor in the complicated social arrangements that made it possible to have children. But you can raise them single-handed now and have sex with lots of different people at the same time. If you've got the energy.

If , however, you decide on a long-term relationship while you're at the family stage, how do you design one that provides a hotbed of sexual excitement and protects the kids as well? Most people still leave it to chance, but deals only work if both sides stick to the contract and that's tricky if there isn't one.

Go through these key criteria with the partner you have in bed or in mind, and see if you both agree about what it's all about.

* **Attractiveness**
  Maybe this is embarrassing to discuss with the person involved, but think it through. If you choose somebody who's prettier than you, you'll need a lot of confidence or power or money to compensate for their beauty. If you choose someone who's less attractive than you, what does that say about your self-esteem? And if you think appearances really don't matter, does your partner agree?

* **Health**

This was more important when survival depended on physical strength. But if the idea is to breed, you might as well go for the best if you have a choice. Maybe you're too blinded by lust to worry about blood tests and too besotted to notice that your partner is drinking and smoking for Britain. But bear in mind that unhealthy habits usually get worse under the pressures of a routine relationship and sleepless nights with a howling baby.

* **Power**
  As Kissinger said, power is the ultimate aphrodisiac. That's why famous but unattractive people often have trophy sex partners. But, famous or not, it's worth checking where the balance of power lies in any relationship. If your partner is more powerful than you in terms of career or charisma, you can have fun redressing the balance in bed – or simply settle for being the wind beneath their wings.

* **Wealth**
Money is sexy too and beauty is often traded for wealth. The advantage of having at least one rich partner in a relationship is being able to afford the trimmings that make sex more fun – like holidays in St Lucia and face-lifts.

* **Emotional factors**
  Do you *like* the person you've selected for long-term sex?

* Write down your separate descriptions of a perfect Sunday. Are they similar?

* List the things you *like* about this person and ask them to do the same about you. It's a bad sign if you can't both get at least eight.

* **Values**
  Dull as they sound, shared values are really important for good, long-term sex. Sit down with your potential partner and make a list of your respective values. If one of you has football at the top followed by work and the other one has family followed by fun, maybe you should just stick with the sex instead of making long-term plans.

Chapter Nine

Income-patibility

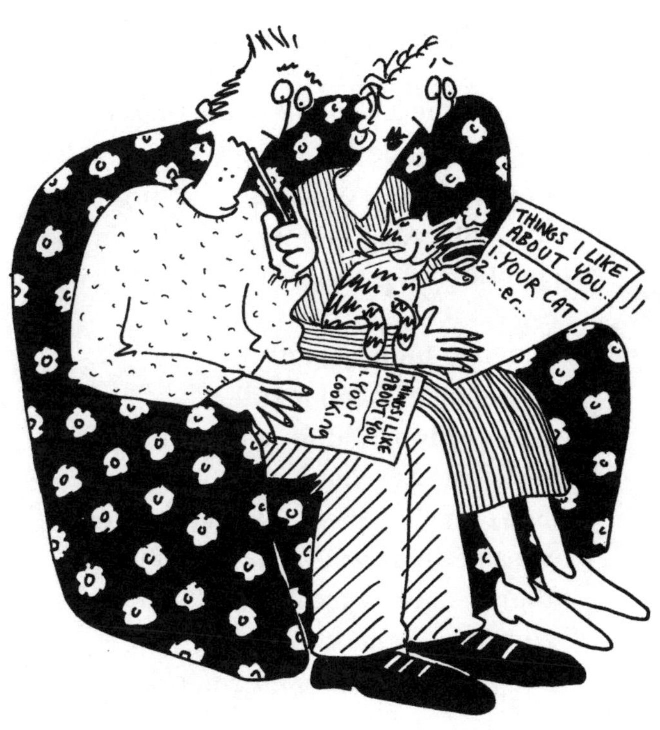

2. The Other Options

If you aren't ready to put in the prep work on a long-term deal you could decide to go for casual sex – or maybe just flirt for a while – until you build up your stamina and confidence again.

* **The one night stand**
  A one night stand is still a relationship. And for a lot of people it's ideal sex – the nearest thing to Erica Jong's 'zipless f***'. Of course it's a pretty recent phenomenon, thanks to birth control and commuting but it's ideal for busy people who don't want emotional

involvement. Unfortunately, low self-esteem is a typical side effect of a one night stand because of the built in Catch 22: 'I don't have to call her again, which is great, but how come she wasn't impressed enough with my performance to call me?'

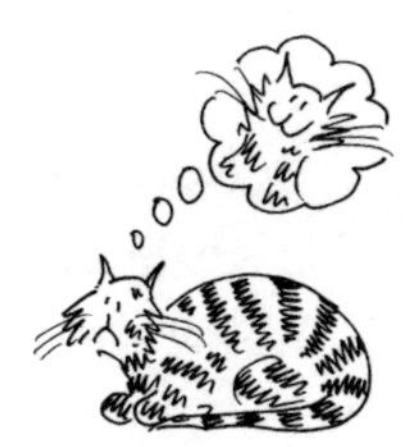

* The accomplished flirt

'You can flirt without having sex, but it's not worth having sex without flirting.'
LORD BELCANNON

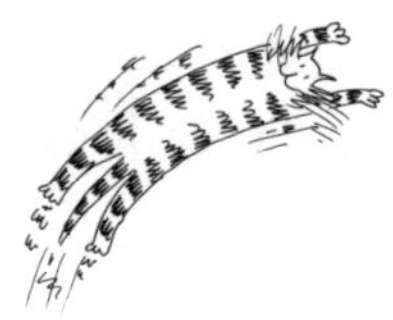

One way of checking out compatibility in advance of commitment is to forget sex for a while and practise flirting instead. Flirting is the ultimate short-term relationship. It's complete in itself, but it's also great practice for the hands-on experience.

Don't expect a result, enjoy the process. Watch the experts around you and learn. People who flirt well do it all the time. Age, sex and inclination make no difference to the accomplished flirt who charms everybody they meet. Flirting is a frame of mind and a very useful one if you want to increase your options for having sex – or improve your chances of having fun.

HOW TO...

* If you are already in bed with somebody, answer as many of these questions together as you can. If that doesn't feel comfortable, maybe you shouldn't be together.

...DO IT

* If you're currently on your own, answer them anyway.

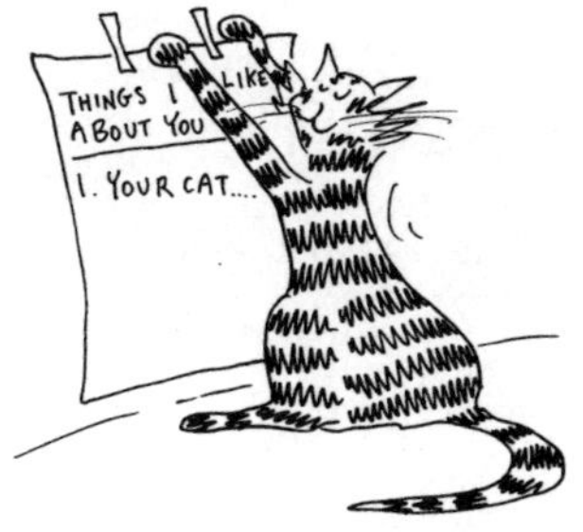
THINGS I LIKE
ABOUT YOU
1. YOUR CAT....

Chapter Ten

What's Love Got To Do With It?

Sex without love is like driving a car with the handbrake on
GEORGES CRUSOE

Love is a ball and chain
CHARLES GERMAINE

BENEFITS

* One small change – a belief about yourself perhaps – can trigger a chain reaction.

BONUS

* The effort you need to make in order to feel an improvement is usually less of an effort than you expect.

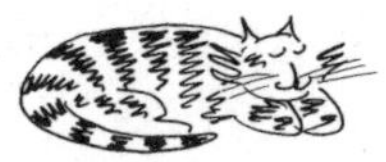

Your sex life will only change if you do. Sex can be either emotional or one-dimensional. If it's just a mechanical exercise, there isn't much you can do, except do it. But when your mind gets involved as well as your body, the brakes are off. Which is great if you're going in the right direction and you don't want to stop.

Sex is a magnet for emotions, but love isn't the only one it attracts. Fear and anger are another couple of front-runners, which is why sex can be dangerous and scary as well as wonderful. So it's a good idea to be picky about the emotions that run your sex life. And, fortunately, you do have a choice.

A lot of people separate emotion and sex completely and, if that doesn't work, they separate sex and other people. Those are both safe options, but not exciting ones. Wouldn't it be nice if you could have emotionally unprotected sex, with no danger of hurting yourself or anyone else?

If that's not been your experience until now, it won't change overnight. However, your deadline for perfect sex probably doesn't have to be as tight as all that, so give yourself some time and start by asking yourself what you could change, whether you really want to change it – and when you're going to start.

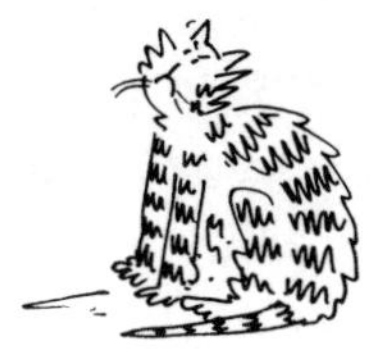

1. The Past

There could be lots of reasons why sex and love haven't been ideal bedmates for you before. Love is one thing and sex is another, but put the two together and you have someone else in your body and mind at the same time. It's a total personal space invasion.

Or maybe you've had a bad experience involving sex in the past. And if you've had one, the chances are you've had several. Traumas travel in convoys like buses, so life may have taught you to disengage your emotions as soon as somebody starts to engage your body. Even if the cause of your detachment was just the negative propaganda about sex that was handed out when you were young, it's surprising how long those messages go on echoing through your brain.

Then again you could be a control freak – and emotional sex is all about being out of control (which is why it's so dangerous if the emotion isn't love).

The reasons don't matter. Once you've identified the problem, you can make a decision not to live with it any more. You can take small positive steps towards doing things differently.

Write down the names of everybody you can remember having sex with in two lists:

GOOD SEX	**BAD SEX**
Name	*Name*
Positive Qualities?	*Positive Qualities?*
Negative Qualities?	*Negative Qualities?*
Length of Relationship?	*Length of Relationship?*
Did you love them?	*Did you love them?*
Did they love you?	*Did they love you?*

The question these questions are helping you to answer is 'has sex been best for me with nice people who love me?' If the answer is No, ask yourself: 'How much do I want to change that? And how am I going to do it?'

Chapter Ten

What's Love Got To Do With It?

You've put ME in the BAD SEX column....!
GOOD SEX
BAD SEX

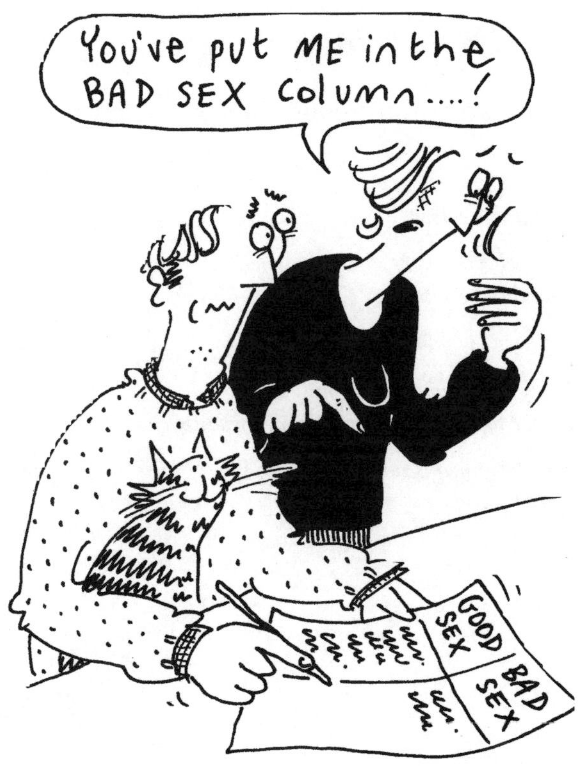

2. The Present

What do you think about sex and love?

Sex is better when excitement, anger or fear are involved.	***Yes / No***
If I love somebody enough, sex with them is bound to be fabulous.	***Yes / No***
If the sex is fabulous, it must be love.	***Yes / No***
If sex with someone is going to be good, I have to fall in love with them instantly.	***Yes / No***
True love means never having to say you're sorry.	***Yes / No***

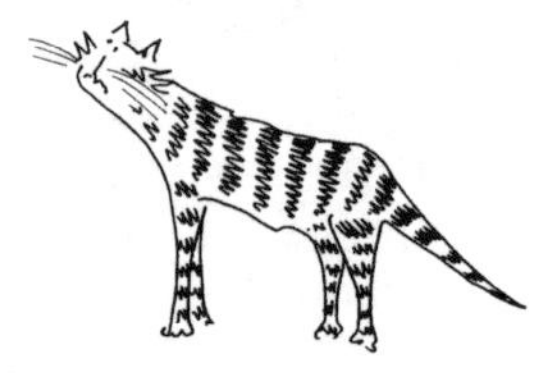

How do you feel about yourself?

I feel lonely when I'm with myself. **Yes / No**

I haven't got much to offer – I need someone to complete me. **Yes / No**

I can't understand why somebody would want a relationship with me. **Yes / No**

I don't usually talk about my feelings. **Yes / No**

I hate talking about other people's feelings. **Yes / No**

If all your answers were *No*, you might as well skip this chapter and go to bed.

But if you mostly answered *Yes*, you're in trouble. High expectations of sex plus low expectations of yourself is a common recipe for a disastrous sex life. So what are you going to do about it?

3. The Future

Which of these things really matter to you? Put a circle round the important ones.

* Appearances: style, fitness, hygiene and eating habits.

* Emotions: warmth, ability to express feelings, closeness to family and friends.

* Social skills: personality and interaction with other people.

* Intellect: education and interests.

* Sex: the ability to enjoy and give pleasure.

* Communication: it doesn't always have to be verbal but it should never be violent. Violence isn't communication; it's communication failure.

* Work and finance: organisational abilities, coping with success and failure and managing money.

* Personal growth potential: willingness to change beliefs and attitudes and work on relationships.

* Interests: innocent pursuits like golf, birdwatching, shopping and football can wreck relationships. Of course, this may really be more to do with values (Chapter Nine).

Check your past relationships against this list to see what worked and what didn't. Then measure up your current partners.

This is the ultimate exercise for change. Not because you need to take this checklist with you every time you meet somebody new, but because it reminds you that you have a right to choose positive loving sex – if that's what you want.

If you use this list to assess potential partners, bear in mind that:

* It doesn't have to be perfect, but it should be positive. People with low self-worth fit neatly with abusive partners. The good thing about abusive relationships is that they don't usually last but the bad thing is that they usually repeat themselves, over and over again. Until somebody changes.

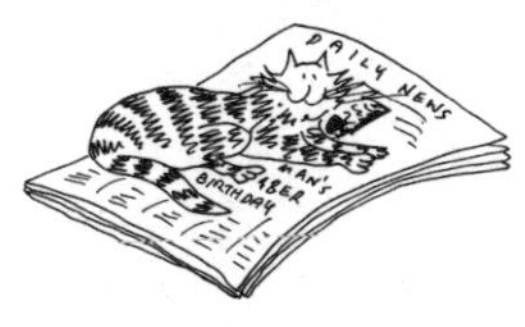

* Don't settle for substitutes. You may think you've found the perfect fit because you like to be cared for and your partner is the nurturing kind – but would your partner be just as happy with a dog or a baby as they are with you? And if they get that dog or that baby, will you suddenly find yourself being neglected?

In other words, have you got a happy future together or just a temporary arrangement?

2. The Happy Ending

This chapter didn't start with a story because the last chapter in a book about you has to be your own story with the ending you want. In Chapter Eight, page 148, I suggested you write an erotic novel, but this time, instead of a fantasy, write your scandalous autobiography, starting from now. Imagine you're looking back on your passionate life after you scrapped your old rules and went back to the emotional drawing board.

If you can't be bothered to write it down, tell it to yourself as a bedtime story every night until you find another way to get off to sleep.

HOW TO...

* Using the Future Checklist gets you into the habit of thinking you have a choice.

...DO IT

* The changes that make a difference are small and manageable, so begin them now. Sidestep one little limiting belief about yourself and take a big step towards better sex.

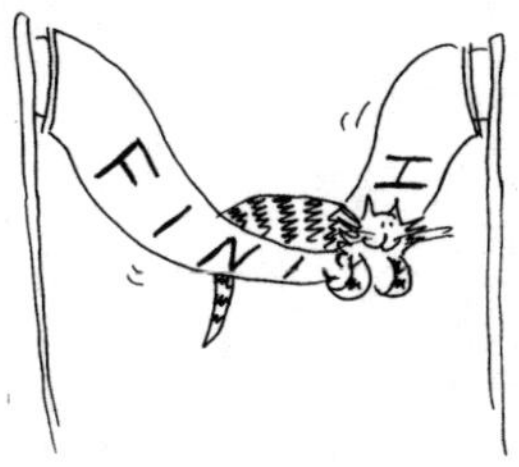
FINI H

Other Books by Judith Verity

Succeeding at Interviews (How To Books)

Feeling Good For No Good Reason (How To Books)

Quick Fix Your Life (How To Books)

Eleven Steps To The User Friendly Office (Bloomsbury)

Lighten Up (Random House)

Slimming With Pete (Crown House)

Doing It With Pete (Crown House)

Titles in the Quick Fix Series

Quick Fix Your Life

Quick Fix Your Emotional Intelligence

Quick Fix Your Web Life